I0025823

WordTOOLS

For

Wellness

Vol. 1

Harnessing the
Power of Words!

Carol L Rickard, LCSW

Well YOUniversity® Publications

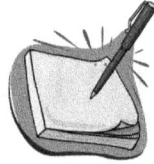

Sign up now!

To be sure to get our weekly motivational &
inspirational quotes and stories!

ThePowerOfWordsEQuote.com

ISBN-13: 978-1-947745-04-9

WordTools for Wellness Vol. 1

Harnessing the Power of Words!

by Carol L Rickard, LCSW

© Copyright 2015 Well YOUniversity Publications

ISBN 13: 978-1-947745-04-9

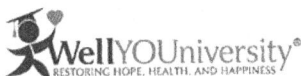

WellYOUniversity®
RESTORING HOPE, HEALTH, AND HAPPINESS

888 LIFE TOOLS (543-3866)

Carol@WellYOUniversity.com

Welcome!

My 1st WordTool came to me in 2006 when doing a group with my patients. How could I get them to *welcome* change in their lives?

Creating **H**ealthy **A**nd **N**ew **G**rowth **E**xperiences!

From there it's been an onward journey! Most of them are inspired by persons or situations. All of them I use in my OWN recovery work. My hope is to create Ah-Ah moments that can help change a life!

They are officially called "Artinyms", which is Sanskrit for "describe".

On the back of each wordtool is a question for you. Answering them will serve to strengthen your wellness.

~To Living Well TODAY! ~

Carol

WordTOOL Guide:

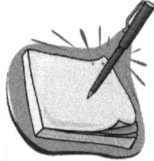

Sign up now!

To be sure to get our weekly motivational &

inspirational quotes and stories!

ThePowerOfWordsEQuote.com

A

Conscious

Choice

Enabling

Powerful

Transformation

What are you are having difficulty *accepting* that could be holding you back? Do you accept you are responsible for your wellness?

A

Critical

Task

Implemented

Only

Now!

What **actions** do you need to take in order to
have more wellness in your life?
What has not taking action cost you?

Awareness

Towards

Thoughts &

Emotions

Needed

To

Improve

Our

Nature

Are there any areas you need to be paying closer **attention** to in order to have more wellness? How about medication, diet, stress?

A

Variation

Only

Increasing

Difficulties

And

Negative

Consequences

Everytime!

In what ways do you tend to *avoid*?

What is something you have been avoiding?

How is that impacting your wellness?

Become

Lost

Amongst

Many

Excuses

When was the last time you **blamed** someone or something instead of owning responsibility? How has blaming hindered your wellness?

Controlling

How

Our

Intention

Creates

Experiences

What are some **choices** you've made that have negatively impacted your wellness?
What are some choices that have helped it?

$\mathbf{C}$onstantly

$\mathbf{H}$aving

$\mathbf{A}$ctivity

$\mathbf{O}$bstruct

$\mathbf{S}$uccess!

What is the *chaos* you need to remove from your life in order to have wellness?
Has chaos stopped you from having wellness?

Concentrate

On

Making

Problems

Larger

Actually

Increasing

Negativity

Make a list of all the things you have been *complaining* about & STOP doing it!

Challenge

Ourselves

Make

Matters

Important

Today!

What is one thing that if you were to **commit** to it would make a huge positive difference in your wellness? What has stopped you?

Don't

Ever

Talk

Excuses

Recognizing

My

Intention

Needs

Exact

Direction

How could your life be different if you become more *determined* to focus on wellness?

Deciding

I

Stay

Committed

In

Purpose

Letting

In

No

Excuses!

What is something you can begin being more *disciplined* about that could improve your wellness? Taking medication, exercise, nutrition?

Daringly

Recognize

Experiences

As

Mine

What would you *dream* to do if you knew you couldn't fail?

Engage

Xternal

Circumstances

Undermining

Self

Empowerment

Who is someone in your life that has empowered you in your journey to wellness?
How did they *empower* you?

Face

An

Important

Lesson

What is the most important lesson you have learned about wellness because you *failed*?

Find

Emotion

Alters

Reality

What has *fear* stopped you from doing?

What would you do if you weren't afraid?

Find

Ourselves

Releasing

Grievances

Including

Victim

Experiences

How do you feel about the word "*forgive*"?

Do you have anyone you cannot forgive?

If so, how does that impact your wellness?

G et

O ur

A ctivity

L ined-up

S traight

What are some of the goals you have for yourself in the next 6 months? Year?
How does wellness impact those goals?

Giving

Respect

And

Thanks

Into

The

Usual

Daily

Experiences

Make a list of 50 things you hold *gratitude*

towards in your life:

(Don't forget little stuff – toothbrush, toilet, etc.)

Having

A

Behavior

Internally

Triggered

What old *habits* are impacting your wellness in a negative way? What new habits do you need to establish to be healthier?

I

Make

Powerful

Adjustments

Concerning

Today

How has not being well impacted your life? What is one thing you could do today to **impact** your health in a positive way?

Leave

Everything

To

God's

Ownership

Do you believe in a higher power as you define it? If so, what things could you *let go* that would have a positive effect on your wellness?

Making

Incremental

Steps

Towards

Achieving

Key

Efforts

What are some of the *mistakes* you have made in the past in regards to your wellness? How have they helped you today?

Natural

Opportunity

To

Inspect

Current

Experiences

When was the last time you took time to notice
the wonderful things around you?

Purposely

Repeat

Activities

Critical

To

Improving

Core

Existence

What are some skills that if you were to *practice* more often could really change your life? What are some of the wellness tools you practice?

Powerful

Underlying

Reason

Push

Ourselves

Stretch

Everyday!

What are the reasons you push yourself to stretch every day? What *purpose* does wellness play in your life?

Re-examine

Experiences

For

Lessons

Enabling

Corrections

Today

What lessons have you learned by *reflecting* on your wellness journey? What do you need to do more of? What do you need to do less of?!

Regain

Every

Characteristic

Of

Value

Empowering

Real

You!

What were some of your strengths before health issues took over your life? What qualities are important to reclaim in your *recovery* journey?

Stop

Old

Behaviors &

Embrace

Recovery

Sober means stopping **ALL HARMFUL behaviors**, not just drugs or alcohol. What are some harmful behaviors you need to stop?

The

Recognizable

Incident

Generating

Great

Emotionally

Response

What are some of your known *triggers*? What impact do they have on your wellness? What triggers do you try to avoid?

$\mathbf{U}$nstoppable

$\mathbf{R}$esponses

$\mathbf{G}$reatly

$\mathbf{E}$ndangering

$\mathbf{S}$elf

What *urges* do you struggle with? Isolation, stress eating, stopping medications?

About the Author

Carol L Rickard, LCSW, TTS, of Hopewell, NJ is founder & CEO of WellYOUniversity, LLC, a global health education company dedicated *to empowering individuals with the tools and supports to achieve lifelong wellness & recovery.*

Also known as ***America's Wellness Ambassador***, Carol is a dynamic & engaging speaker who brings to life practical / useful solutions. She is a weekly contributor for Esperanza Magazine; written 13 books on stress and wellness, had a guest appearance on Dr. Oz last year

She is also the creator & host of a 30-minute wellness show on Princeton TV - **The WELL YOU Show** which current episodes are aired on Mondays at 6:00pm EST & Sundays at 8:30am EST and can be watched at PrincetonTV.org.

All episodes available at: **www.TheWELLYOUShow.com**

Get more of Carol at:

Twitter: ***@wellYOUlife***

"Like us" @ www.FaceBook.com/WellYOUniversity

Have Carol Speak at Your Next Event!

Get more information about how you can have Carol speak at your organization, event, or conference.

Go to: www.CarolLRickard.com

Or call: 888 Life Tools (543-3866)

Carol's Other Books

Getting Your Mind to Mind You

ANGER – A Simple & Practical Approach

Help – How to Help Those Who DON'T Want it

Selfness – Simple Self-Care Secrets

Stress Eating – How to STOP Using Food to Cope

Stretched Not Broken – Caregiver's Stress

The Caregiver's Toolbox

Transforming Illness to Wellness

Putting Your Weight Loss on Auto

The Benefits of Smoking

Moving Beyond Depression

LifeTools – How to Manage Life

Creating Compliance

Relapse Prevention

Please visit us at:

www.WellYOUniversity.com

Sign up for weekly motivational e-quote!

Check out our upcoming FREE webinars!

Learn more about our training programs.

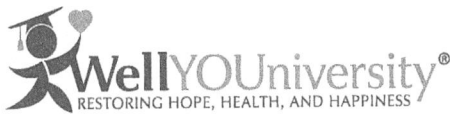

WellYOUniversity®
RESTORING HOPE, HEALTH, AND HAPPINESS

Email us your success story at:

Success@WellYOUniversity.com

We'd like to ask for your feedback

Please check out the next page
if this book has been HELPFUL for you!

We'd love to hear from you!

Feedback Card

Please take a moment & provide us some

feedback about the book you just read &

how you feel *it benefited YOU!*

_____

_____

_____

_____

Name: _____

Best Phone #: _____

Can we use your comments in our publicity materials?

Yes / No

If OK with you, what's the best time to call you:_____

Thank You!

Scan or take a picture & email:

Carol@WellYOUniversity.com

Snail mail: Carol Rickard

5 Zion Rd., Hopewell, NJ 08535

www.ingramcontent.com/pod-product-compliance
Lightning Source LLC
Chambersburg PA
CBHW070931280326
41934CB00009B/1834